SEX BOOSTERS

Spice Up Your Sex Life with Natural Aphrodisiacs!

By James Adler

Copyright James Adler© 2014, 2016

All rights reserved. No part of this publication may be reproduced, stored in a retrieval system, or transmitted, in any form or by any means, electronic, mechanical, photocopying, recording or otherwise, without the prior written permission of the author and the publishers.

The scanning, uploading, and distribution of this book via the Internet or via any other means without the permission of the author is illegal and punishable by law. Please purchase only authorized electronic editions, and do not participate in or encourage electronic piracy of copyrighted materials.

Disclaimer:

A physician has not written the information in this book. Although natural and herbal treatments are generally safe to use, if you suffer from any serious medical condition, are pregnant, or on medication you should consult your physician first to see if you can apply the natural remedies described in this book. It is also advisable that you visit your local herbalist so that you can obtain a highly personalized treatment for your case. Most of the natural remedies can be safely employed at the same time but it is still always recommended to consult your physician first. Before you start using any of the herbal treatments recommended in this book, please get acquainted with possible contra indications (especially if you are on medication) and research the brand.

Table of Contents

Chapter 1 Aphrodisiac Foods 11
Recipes 15
Recipe Measurements 17
Libido Boosting Avocado with Shrimp 18
Carribean Dream Libido Boosters 22
Delicious Oyster Libido Boosting Snacks 24
Mediterrean Mushrooms 26
Quinoa Aphrodisiac Dessert 28
Strawberry & Chocolate Libido Stimulating Dream 30
Aphrodisiac Apple Cream 32
Fresh Libido Stimulating Fruit Salad 34
Sexy Prawns 35
Aphrodisiac Mayo Dressing 37
Super Easy & Libido Stimulating Orange Salad 38
Raw Aphrodisiac Candies 39
Libido Stimulating Raw Chocolate Dip 41
Chapter 2 Aphrodisiac Drinks 42
PART I: Alcoholic Beverages - Romantic Dinners ... 43
Matahari 43
Secret Crush 44
Fraise Sauvage 45

Malena 46
Chai Infused Sweet Vermouth 47
Aphrodisiac Gin & Tonic for Special Occasions...... 48
Spanish "Tinto Del Verano" Summertime Libido Booster.. 49
Alcohol Free Aphrodisiac Cocktail 50
Amazing Libido Stimulating Pink Smoothie 51
Aphrodisiac Choco Smoothie with Guarana.............52
Super Magnesium Power Smoothie 54
Coconut Alkaline Aphrodisiac Exotic Smoothie.......55
Carrot Aphrodisiac Power 57
Chapter 4 Aphrodisiac Herbs 59
Chapter 5 Aromatherapy 76
Massage Techniques For Lovers............................... 93

Introduction

Thank you for taking interest in my book. It really means a lot to me and I sincerely hope that you and your partner will find it useful.

I have decided to create this book in order to inspire you and give you some practical tools and solutions so that you can improve your sex life with your partner. As a bonus, I have also included plenty of amazingly delicious recipes for romantic dinners and other libido stimulating meals. My recipes are quick to prepare - perfect for busy people in the 21st century.

I hope that some of the natural aphrodisiacs that I mention in this little book, even if not new to you, will take your sex life to a whole new level. Females and males are different creatures and so it is obvious that aphrodisiacs recommended may also differ. Some of the natural 'sex boosters' work better for men, some of them work better for women. All of my research and my personal experiences are included in this book.

Now...let's try to spice it up!

The human touch is used universally to communicate feelings. It is evident throughout history, arts and even legends that humans have an inevitable need to express deep emotions through physical intimacy.

The word aphrodisiac is inspired by the Greek goddess of love, Aphrodite, who as the legend describes, has the ability to stimulate desire and promote sexuality. Cleopatra is among the notable women who used aphrodisiac to their advantage. This seductress is said to have used oil and perfume derived from flowers to captivate her lovers.

Benefits of using Natural Sex Boosters:

You might think that pleasure is the only benefit derived from aphrodisiacs but surprisingly, natural aphrodisiacs have other health benefits as well:

-Some aphrodisiacs improve blood circulation and can even prevent high blood pressure.

-Having more sex works as a powerful antioxidant that helps keep your hormones in check.

-Having sex regularly reduces the stress hormones in the body by triggering the pleasure centers of the brain.

-Another popular reason for indulging in aphrodisiacs is that it helps to maintain a healthy body weight. Most people would naturally feel more motivated to have sex than go to the gym. What's more fun for you?

Finally, is there anything better than making passionate love to someone you love and have a special connection with?

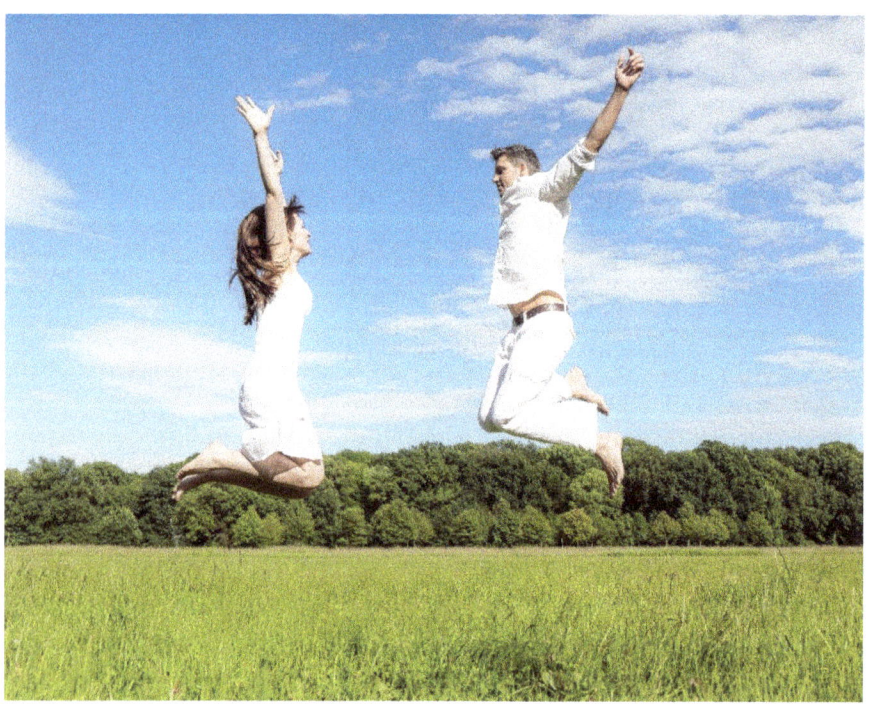

Why Natural?

I would like to make you realize that utilizing natural aphrodisiacs (foods, recipes, herbs, aromatherapy and massage) is not only about getting a new, natural quick fix. It's about embracing a new, healthy and balanced lifestyle and adapting it to your personal needs.

Many people prefer quick fixes like taking some libido boosting pills. Such solutions are short-term. What I describe here, in this book is a myriad of natural solutions that will help you and your partner create new libido boosting rituals. Yes, new, sexy rituals. As a result, you will be able to develop more empathy and a better connection with each other.

Remember to respect your partner - this is rule number one. Communication is the most important thing in a relationship. Never force your partner into doing something they don't feel like doing. Use natural aphrodisiacs and share them with your partner only if they agree to it. Some herbal remedies may interact with standard medications and other conditions, so never offer any of those to your partner without their knowledge.

Free Complimentary eBook + Health Newsletter

Before we dive into the amazing world of natural aphrodisiacs, I would like to offer you a free complimentary PDF eBook:

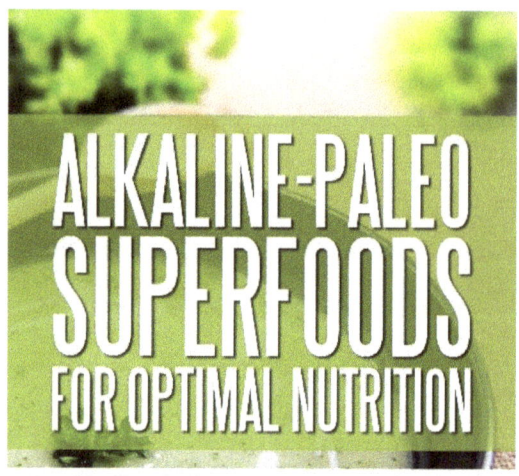

Download link:

www.holisticwellnessbooks.com/bonus

Problems with your download?

Contact us: elenajamesbooks@gmail.com

Chapter 1 Aphrodisiac Foods

For centuries, humans believed that anything that resembles the genitals (as weird as it sounds!) can possess sexual powers. Sea food, vegetables and spices are the common traditional aphrodisiac foods found in different cultures.

Try these aphrodisiac foods to boost your appetite for some bedroom action:

Oysters

The Ancient Romans believed that oysters are the most powerful and effective aphrodisiac there is. I recommend eating oysters raw which is best served with crushed ice and seaweed. The legendary Casanova was also a fan of oysters and had the habit of eating 50 raw oysters every morning with the lady he fancied.

Scientifically speaking, oysters are low in fat and high in zinc which is said to increase sperm and testosterone levels in the body.

Onion

Onions are mentioned in classic Hindu texts as an aphrodisiac and were included in many Greek and Roman recipes as sexual stimulants. In Ancient Egypt, celibate priests were even forbidden to eat onions because of their sexual effects. Arab folklore suggests pounding onion and mixing it with honey to achieve better results (might be a good idea to mix the two ingredients in a salad, right?).

Truffles

Truffles are expensive fungi that have a pungent odor, but are also known as a potent aphrodisiac. The scent of truffles is said to mimic that of andostenone which attracts the opposite sex. During the Roman times, Libyan truffles were considered to be the highest rated truffle; however, its popularity grew weak and was only rediscovered during the eighteenth century in France.

Asparagus

The shape of asparagus is said to be a symbol of its aphrodisiac qualities. I recommend boiling the asparagus and frying it with some healthy fat (coconut oil or olive oil) to enhance its properties.

However, while asparagus can be sexually stimulating for men, it has the opposite effect on women.

Celery

Celery has a long history of being used as an aphrodisiac. Its stalks can be eaten raw. Celery is a popular aphrodisiac in Poland and Czech Republic. Take note that boiling celery can reduce its sexual benefits.

Carrots

Based on Ukrainian belief, carrots have great aphrodisiac effects especially for men who have lost their sexual vigor.

Coco-de Mer

Coco de-mer is not only visually stimulating because of its close resemblance to a female body part but it also acts as an aphrodisiac when consumed.

The annual production for coco-de mer is only limited to a few thousand per year, so you can eat coconut instead and still achieve similar results.

Quince

Quince was called as the golden apple of Hesperides which is a symbol for sexuality in Greece. Due to its color and fragrance, it has been dedicated to the goddess of love and was used as a symbol of fertility and happy marriage.

Coriander

Coriander was used as an aphrodisiac in the story of Arabian Nights. The coriander's warming properties are the likely source of its aphrodisiac qualities. Sprinkle ground coriander in soups and even salads as much as you can.

Piranha

Piranhas are carnivorous fish that reside in the rivers of Central and South America. In Brazil, Piranha soup is believed to have invigorating properties that can boost a flagging sexual stamina.

Honey

Organic raw honey enhances testosterone production and increases sexual desire in men. It also has Boron which is essential in estrogen production. Use honey as your main sweetener and feel the aphrodisiac effect that it gives.

Chili peppers

Chili heats up the body and encourages blood flow. Eating spicy food also gives you an appearance that is suggestive of sexual desire, such as flushed skin and swollen lips. Chili peppers have been used for centuries because of their ability to produce feel-good hormones.

Green, alkaline veggies

These foods help balance your pH and, if consumed regularly, will help you boost your energy naturally. Green veggies are also excellent natural antioxidants. Add more spinach, avocados, kale, cucumbers and carrots into your diet. Radish, onions and garlic are also extremely alkaline. Alternatively, you can use green powders and supplements (Make sure you research the brand. I use Doctor Young's products if you need a recommendation).

PRACTICAL PART- RECIPES

Of course, it's not about just snacking on these foods. One needs to learn how to create amazing, nutritious, libido-stimulating mouth-watering dishes. This is why I am sharing some of my favorite recipes that my wife and I have tested dozens of times!

It's time for some romantic cooking...

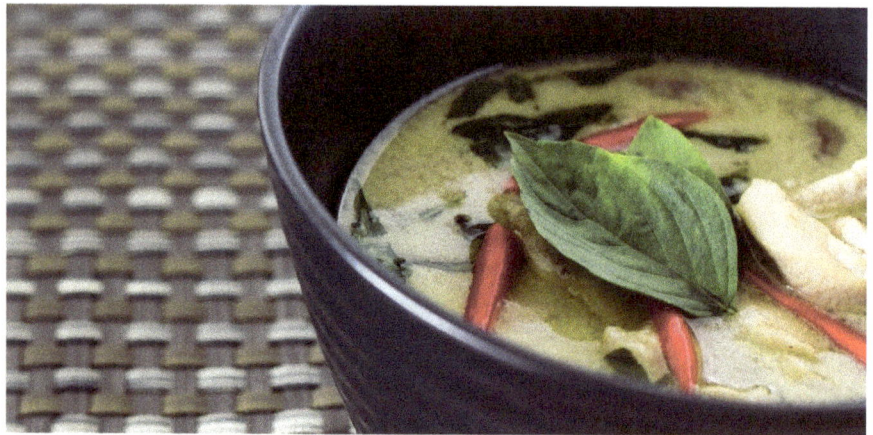

Recipe Measurements

I love keeping ingredient measurements as simple as possible- this is why I stick to tablespoons, teaspoons and cups.

The cup measurement I use is the American cup measurement. I also use it for dry ingredients. If you are new to it, let me help you:

If you don't have American Cup measures, just use a metric or imperial liquid measuring jug and fill your jug with your ingredient to the corresponding level. Here's how to go about it:

1 American Cup= 250ml= 8 fl.oz

For example:

If a recipe calls for 1 cup of almonds, simply place your almonds into your measuring jug until it reaches the 250 ml/8oz mark.

I know that different countries use different measurements and I wanted to make things simple for you.

AMAZING LIBIDO BOOSTING (PALEO-INSPIRED) AVOCADO WITH SHRIMP

Serves-2

Ingredients

- 2 avocados
- pink sauce (you can also use mustard)
- ½ cup of peeled and cooked prawns
- 2 fresh oysters
- Lemon juice
- 1 head of lettuce
- 1 tomato, chopped
- 1 onion, minced
- Pinch of chili powder
- ½ cup smoked salmon
- Himalayan salt (this salt is actually good for you, it contains iron and magnesium)

Instructions:

1. Prepare avocados and cut into halves.
2. Cut the salmon and lettuce leaves into strips, season with cocktail sauce and a pinch of black pepper to taste.
3. Place the lettuce and salmon on a big plate. Season it with olive oil, lemon juice and some Himalaya salt

4. Place avocado halves on top of the salad.
5. In a bowl, mix tomato (chopped), shrimp, pink salsa and onions. Add chili powder and Himalayan salt.
6. Place the mixture on top of each avocado half.
7. Place the oysters next to each avocado half.

APHRODISIAC BASMATI RICE
Serves-2

Ingredients:

- 2 Cups of basmati rice
- 8 cups water
- 2 large coconuts (you can also use 1-2 cups of fresh coconut milk, so yummy!)
- 2 cups of shrimp
- 2 cups of squid
- 1 lobster
- 15 Crab claws
- 1 big bell pepper
- 2 onions
- 4 cloves of garlic
- Oil, salt and pepper
- 1 tablespoon achiote (Bixa orellana). You can also use other spices

Preparation:

1. Grate the coconut and add four cups of boiling water. Squeeze well to extract milk, and set aside.

2. Clean and cut the squid, shrimp and lobster.

3. Fry the chopped onion and crushed garlic in some olive or coconut oil. Reserve.

4. In the same pan you have just used, fry the pepper and add the coconut milk with water, letting it simmer.

5. Bring to a boil, add the seafood and rice and cook until rice is done.

6. Just before removing the fire (few minutes before), add the remaining sauce (onions and garlic from step 3).

7. Enjoy☺

CARRIBEAN DREAM LIBIDO BOOSTERS

Fruits are full of vitamins and minerals. Some people worry about high sugar content, but guess what...? You can burn it off in your bedroom!

Serves- 2-4

Ingredients:

- 2 ripe bananas (sliced and cooled down in a freezer for about 30 mins.)
- Half mango, chopped
- 2 cups of pineapple chunks
- 2 tablespoons of cinnamon
- 1 tablespoon of ginger (powdered)
- 1 teaspoon lemon juice
- 1 teaspoon lime juice
- 2 tablespoons of Jamaican rum
- 1 cup of coconut milk (can be also rice milk or almond milk, we love coconut milk though)
- 2 tablespoons of coconut oil

- Half cup of soaked agar-agar seaweed
- 2 tablespoons chopped almonds
- Raw, organic honey or cane sugar to taste

Preparation:

1. Mix all the ingredients in a big bowl.
2. Put in a fridge for about 1 hour. Enjoy!
3. Place in 2 separate bowls (or use one if you wish to share) and pour over some Jamaican rum before serving.
4. Enjoy!

DELICIOUS OYSTER LIBIDO BOOSTING SNACKS (QUICK PREP).

Serves-2

Ingredients:

- A few integral rice cakes or a few gluten free crackers
- 12 oysters
- A few onion rings
- A few slices of tomato
- A few avocado slices
- Coconut oil
- chives
- lemon
- pepper to taste
- chili power to taste
- a few lemon slices

Instructions:

1. Smear each rice cake with coconut oil.

2. Place an avocado slice/ tomato slice and onion ring on each rice cake. Add oysters.

3. Sprinkle over some chili powder, lemon juice and pepper to taste and spice it up.

4. Garnish with a few lemon slices.

5. Enjoy!

MEDITERREAN MUSHROOMS
Serves-2

Ingredients:

- Pinch of savory
- Pinch of parsley
- Pinch of cilantro
- Half lemon
- 1 onion, minced
- 2 garlic cloves, minced
- Salt
- pepper
- 1 cup of mushrooms
- 1/2 cup of olive oil

Preparation:

1. Fry onion and garlic in olive oil. Stop the heat when they start to brown. Set aside on a plate.
2. Add the spices and the mushrooms to the pan. Keep

adding more oil and water and stir fry over medium heat.

3. Add the onions & garlic.

4. Stir well and keep on low heat for a few mins. Stop the heat. Add a bit of lemon juice before serving.

Enjoy! So delicious!

We love to serve it with quinoa (also a great aphrodisiac and really healthy) or amaranth (another aphrodisiac grain).

You can cook quinoa or amaranth grains and store them in your freezer. Quinoa is gluten-free and an excellent source of natural protein. The following recipe will help you prepare quinoa libido stimulating dessert…

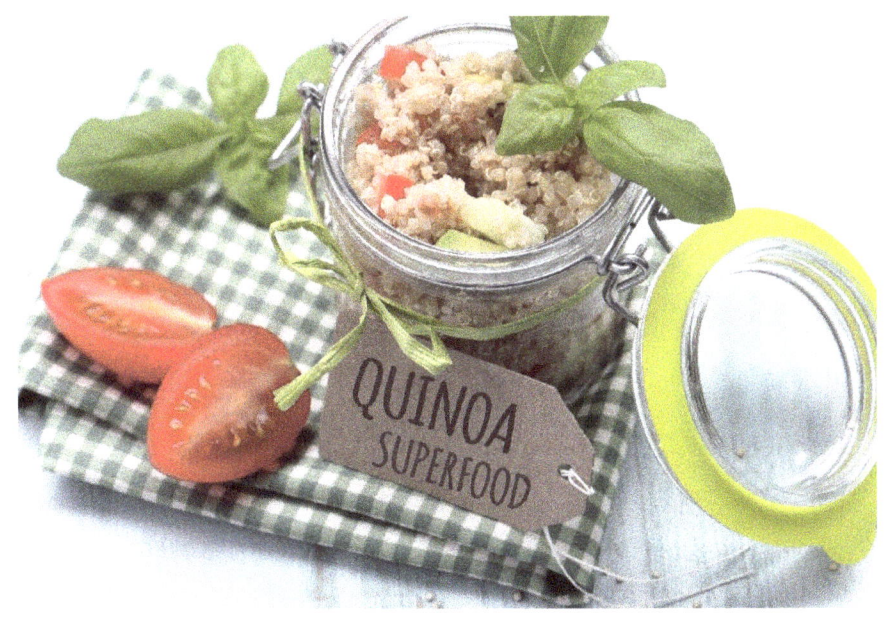

QUINOA APHRODISIAC DESSERT

Serves-2

Ingredients:

- 2 cups of cooked quinoa
- 1 cup of coconut milk
- 2 tablespoons of rum (optional) or Bailey's Irish Cream
- 2 tablespoons of raw honey or cane sugar
- 1 cup of strawberries, sliced
- Half cup of raisins
- 2 tablespoons of cinnamon
- A few cherries to garnish
- A bit of cream to garnish (I recommend coconut cream)

Preparation:

1. In a big bowl, mix quinoa, coconut milk, rum, honey, strawberries and raisins.
2. Place in a fridge for about 30 mins.
3. Serve in dessert glasses. Garnish with some cream and

cherries on top.

4. Enjoy!

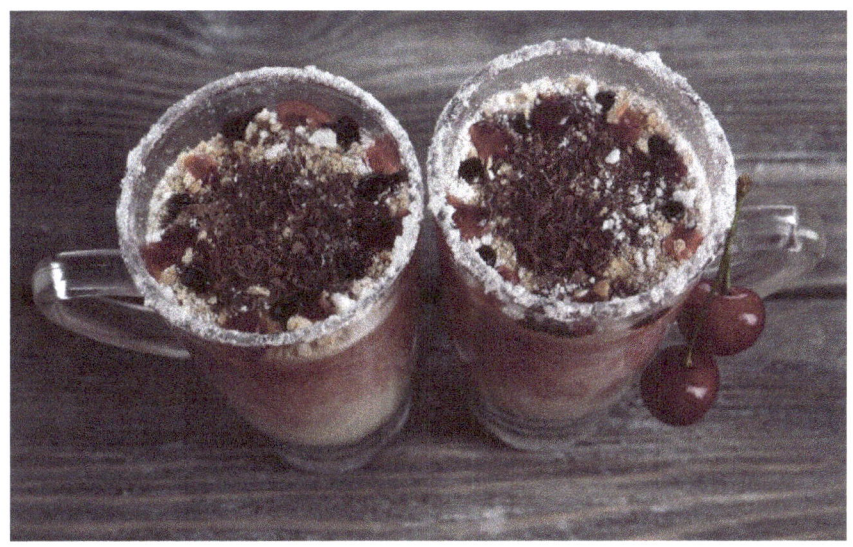

STRAWBERRY AND CHOCLATE LIBIDO STIMULATING DREAM

I find this dessert absolutely amazing!

Serves- 2

Ingredients:

- 1 cup of whole strawberries
- 2 cups of almond milk
- 5 tablespoons of cocoa powder (organic)
- 2 tablespoons vanilla
- Cinnamon to season

Preparation:

1. Bring almond milk to boil.
2. Add cocoa powder and a bit of cinnamon and vanilla.
3. Turn off the heat when boiling; make sure there are no lumps of cocoa powder.
4. Place the strawberries in a bowl.
5. Pour cocoa drink over the strawberries.

6. Place in a fridge for a few hours.

7. Serve chilled!

8. Enjoy!

APHRODISIAC APPLE CREAM

I love apples! As they say, an apple a day will keep a doctor away. Plus, we can spice things up....

Serves-2

Ingredients:

- 4 big apples
- Half cup of coconut milk
- 2 tablespoons of sesame powder
- 1 tablespoon of cinnamon
- 1 cup of cherries
- 2 tablespoons of rum
- 1 cup of raisins
- 2 bananas

Preparation:

1. Wash, peel, and chop the apples, remove the seeds. Place in blender.
2. Blend apples with coconut milk, bananas and raisins.

3. Add cinnamon and juice of 1 lemon with rum. Stir well and refrigerate for 1 hour.

4. Pour in 2 dessert glasses, sprinkle over some sesame powder (it's great for natural energy) and add cherries on top..So amazing and libido stimulating!

FRESH LIBIDO STIMULATING FRUIT SALAD

I love fruit and could not live without it. Adding fresh, organic fruit into your diet, will make you more energetic and fit. All we need, right?

Serves-2

Ingredients:

- arugula leaves (1/2 cup)
- half cup strawberry, sliced
- 2 kiwis, peeled and chopped
- 1 tablespoon balsamic vinegar.
- Cane Sugar
- Ground black pepper
- Lime juice

Preparation:

1. Mix all the ingredients in a big bowl.
2. Sprinkle over some lime juice and vinegar. Serve.

SEXY PRAWNS

Serves-2

Ingredients:

- 2 cups of peeled and washed prawns
- Pinch of powdered red pepper
- 2 bay leaves
- 1 teaspoon salt
- Half a cup of olive oil
- 1 cup wine vinegar
- 3 cloves garlic, minced
- 1 tablespoon spices to taste

Ingredients:

1. Boil all ingredients except shrimp for 2 minutes.
2. Add the shrimp and cook for about 3 minutes.
3. Remove from the heat. Cool down in a fridge.
4. Serve cold.

MY TIP

You can mix them with chopped avocados, radishes and tomatoes. So delicious and aphrodisiac!

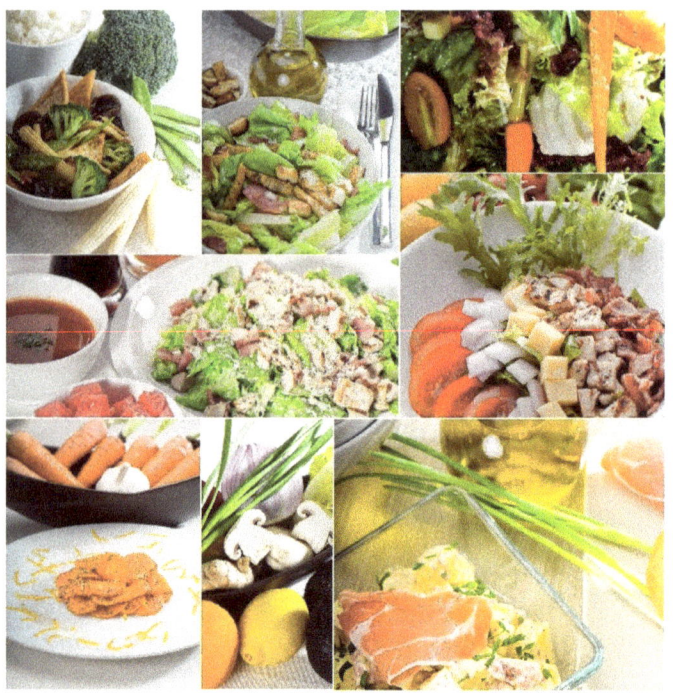

APHRODISIAC MAYO DRESSING

Ingredients:

- egg yolk
- mustard
- pinch of thyme, sage, basil, rosemary
- teaspoon of chili powder and salt

Mix all the ingredients in a small bowl. Save in a fridge for at least 1 hour. Perfect to serve with salmon and seafood, as well as salads dressing.

Remember to grab your free recipe ebook:

www.holisticwellnessbooks.com/bonus

SUPER EASY & LIBIDO STIMULATING ORANGE SALAD

Pressed for time? Looking for a quick and healthy aphrodisiac snack to share with your partner?

Serves-2

Ingredients:

- 4 oranges, peeled and sliced
- ¼ cup of crushed mint
- 2 teaspoons grated ginger
- 2 tablespoons of olive oil
- a pinch of Himalayan salt
- black pepper to taste

Preparation:

Mix all the ingredients in a bowl. Serve immediately!

RAW APHRODISIAC CANDIES (QUICK PREP)

I am absolutely in love with this healthy, raw treat!

Serves- as many as you need!

Ingredients:

- 1 cup tahini
- 3 cups honey,
- 1 teaspoon cinnamon,
- 1 teaspoon ginger,
- 1 teaspoon anise and cardamom,
- 2 tablespoons cocoa,
- vanilla essence to taste,
- grated coconut.
- Optional: tablespoon mint leaves into small pieces.

Preparation:

1. Mix sesame paste with honey.
2. Add vanilla, cinnamon, anise, cardamom and ginger.
3. Form small balls.
4. Roll them in cocoa and grated coconut.
5. Cool in refrigerator for about half an hour and serve.
6. Enjoy!

LIBIDO STIMULATING RAW CHOCLATE DIP (QUICK PREP)

Makes 1 cup

Ingredients:

- 5 tablespoons of cocoa powder (raw and organic)
- 1 big banana
- 1 cup of coconut milk
- 2 tablespoons of raw honey or cane sugar
- Coconut oil and almond powder to achieve desired consistency (it's up to you)

Preparation:

1. Blend all the ingredients.
2. Store in a fridge for at least a few hours.
3. Serve with fresh fruit; for example, cherries (sexy!) or strawberries.
4. Enjoy!

Chapter 2 Aphrodisiac Drinks

Aphrodisiac drinks can stimulate sexual desire and take your relationship to a new level. I have included alcoholic beverages as well as juices and smoothies. Pick up whatever suits you and your partner and, of course, your occasion. It might be a romantic dinner, or simply the urge to stimulate your libido during the day. Alcohol can be helpful but only occasionally and in small amounts. I totally recommend you use natural smoothies and juices as much as possible as they will add to your overall wellness and health. This is the most important thing if you wish to remain sexually fit and attractive. It all comes down to creating new, healthy habits and sticking to them on a regular basis.

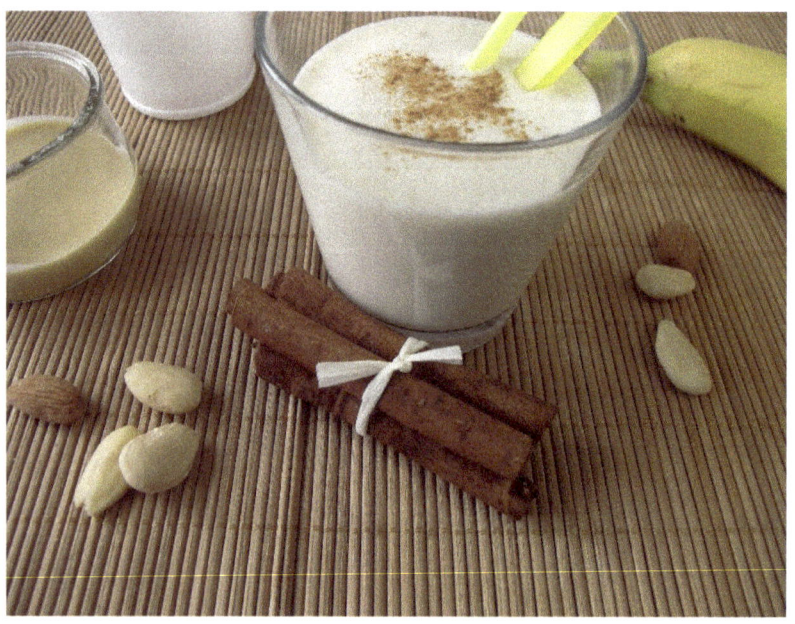

PART I: ALCOHOLIC BEVERAGES FOR ROMANTIC DINNERS

Matahari

The Matahari drink is named after one of the greatest femme fatales in human history. Matahari is a drink that has exotic flavors and it also comes in many colors.

Serves-2

Ingredients:

- 1 oz Chai-infused Vermouth
- 1 ¼ oz Pierre Ferrand Amber Cognac

½ oz simple syrup

- lemon juice (1 tablespoon)
- ¾ oz Pomegranate juice
- 3 dried organic rose buds

Preparation:

1. Shake ingredients (except rose buds) energetically with ice.
2. Pour into cocktail glasses and use rose buds as garnish.

SECRET CRUSH

The secret crush is a variation of champagne cocktail. This cocktail drink is a very sexy and inviting drink that is best paired with seafood appetizers.

Serves-2

Ingredients:

- ¾ oz Campari
- 5 oz Llopart Cava Leopardi Brut Rose
- 2 brown sugar cubes
- 4-5 dashes of Angostura bitters
- 1 lemon twist

Preparation:

1. Pour half of the wine into a champagne flute and place the sugar cube on a bar spoon.
2. Saturate the mixture with Angostura Bitters and add sugar cube. Let it rest for a few minutes and then pour in the rest of the wine.
3. Add Campari and a very small amount of pearl dust.
4. Garnish with a lemon twist.

FRAISE SAUVAGE

Fraise Sauvage is a cocktail that is inspired by the famous French 75, a drink that is named after the French 75 mm caliber artillery guns. Despite its masculine origin, this aphrodisiac drink uses strawberries as its main ingredient.

Serves-2

Ingredients:

- 1 ¼ oz Tanqueray Gin
- ¼ oz simple syrup
- ½ oz fresh lemon juice
- ¾ cup Strawberry puree
- 2 oz Prossecco
- Half strawberry for garnish

Preparation:

1. Pour all the ingredients except the Prossecco into a mixing glass and add ice before shaking vigorously for few seconds.
2. Pour the Prossecco into a cocktail glass before pouring the cocktail over it. Garnish with the strawberry.

MALENA

Malena is a fantastic drink that pays homage to Negroni Nirvana. Malena is a delicious drink but it can also be addicting. The bold and bitter-sweet taste of malena is what makes it a seductive aphrodisiac.

Serves-2

Ingredients:

- 1 oz Campari
- 1 oz Rittenhouse Straight Rye Whiskey
- ¾ oz Ruby Port
- 6 grapes
- 3 dash of orange bitters
- A few drops of orange blossom water
- Ground cinnamon
- 2 slices of orange to garnish

Preparation:

1. Mix all the ingredients and add ice.
2. Sprinkle little bit of cinnamon and garnish with a slice of orange. Enjoy!

CHAI INFUSED SWEET VERMOUTH

Chai has intoxicating flavor properties. When combined with sweet vermouth, it produces an exotic tasting cocktail.

Serves-2

Ingredients:

- 8 green cardamom pods
- 1 cinnamon stick
- 8 cloves
- 1 inch ginger coarsely chopped
- 2 tbsp chai
- 2 liters sweet vermouth

Preparation:

1. Place the cinnamon, cloves and cardamom into a saucepan and heat for 1 minute.
2. Add the chai and 2 cups of vermouth.
3. Turn off the heat. Wait until the mix cools down.
4. Add vermouth and pour the mix into a bottle. Cool down in a fridge. Serve cold, enjoy!

APHRODISIAC GIN AND TONIC FOR SPECIAL OCCASIONS

Serves 2

Ingredients:

- 2 shots of Bombay Sapphire gin
- 10 strawberries, sliced
- A few mint leaves
- Lots of ice
- Tonic water

Preparation:

1. Mix all the ingredients.
2. Add strawberry slices and ice.
3. Garnish with a slice of lime.
4. Enjoy and remember to drink in moderation!

SPANISH "TINTO DEL VERANO" SUMMERTIME LIBIDO BOOSTER

I love this drink on hot summers!

Serves 2 or more

Ingredients:

- Half a liter of red wine
- Half a liter of soda
- Red Martini
- Juice of 1 lime
- 1 lemon
- Ice

Preparation:

1. Pour ice and wine into a large vessel.
2. Add a dash of Martini Red (to taste).
3. Fill the rest of the way with soda and lime juice.
4. Garnish with a few slices of lemon. Serve cold.

ALCOHOL FREE APHRODISIAC COCKTAIL

Ingredients (2 serves):

- 1 cup of fresh orange juice
- 2 egg yolks
- 4 teaspoons of coconut milk
- 2 teaspoons honey
- Cinnamon
- Ice cubes
- Lemon slices to garnish

Preparation:

1. Blend all the ingredients.
2. Pour into a glass.
3. Serve with a slice of lemon and more ice cubes if you wish.

AMAZING LIBIDO STIMULATING PINK SMOOTHIE

Serves-2

Ingredients

- 4 mandarins
- 2 cups of raspberries
- 1 cup of blueberries
- 2 apples
- 1 cup of almond milk
- 1 cup of coconut milk
- 2 tablespoons of coconut oil for more consistency
- 2 teaspoons of maca powder

Preparation:

1. Blend all ingredients and enjoy!
2. Serve immediately.

HEALTHY APHRODISIAC CHOCO SMOOTHIE WITH GUARANA

Be careful, this smoothie is extremely powerful!

Before using guarana, make sure that it is suitable for you. People who are caffeine sensitive, have high blood pressure, or are on medication should refrain from using guarana. As always, I suggest you consult your physician first. The same applies to maca powder - some people may experience nausea and headaches as well as digestive issues, so make sure it is safe for you. You don't want to spoil your night, right?

Serves-2

Ingredients:

- 2 bananas
- 2 avocados
- 1 tablespoon of cinnamon
- 4 tablespoons of dark, organic cocoa powder
- 2 cups of almond milk
- 1 teaspoon of guarana or maca powder

Instructions:

Blend and enjoy!

OPTIONAL: you can also add some green alkaline powder to your smoothie. I recommend it for those who can't use maca or guarana. Alfalfa powder is an excellent option. It is extremely alkaline and energizing plus it does wonders for hair and skin (natural beauty treatment that my wife is a big fan of!).

Remember to grab your free recipe eBook:

www.holisticwellnessbooks.com/bonus

SUPER MAGNESIUM POWER SMOOTHIE

Serves-2

Ingredients:

- 2 bananas
- 1 mango
- 2 cups of rice milk
- 1 cup of espresso, cooled
- Ice cubes

Preparation:

Blend all the ingredients. Coffee gives it a nice taste and stimulation. Full power!

COCONUT 100% ALKALINE APHRODISIAC EXOTIC SMOOTHIE

I am absolutely in love with this spicy and exotic smoothie. When talking about alkaline smoothies, many people think that it's probably all green and tasteless. Well, check out this one. All the ingredients are super alkaline and will give you and your partner an amazing energy boost! Moreover, its amazing fragrance is also libido stimulating and extremely relaxing (more on fragrances in the aromatherapy section of this book).

Serves-2

Ingredients:

- 2 tablespoons of ginger powder
- 1 tablespoon of nutmeg
- 1 teaspoon of cinnamon
- 1 teaspoon of clove
- 2 cups of coconut milk
- 1 avocado
- Juice of 2 limes

OPTIONAL:

- 1 teaspoon of maca powder

- 1 tablespoon of green, alkaline powder (highly recommended!)

Instructions:

Blend and enjoy! Serve with some ice cubes.

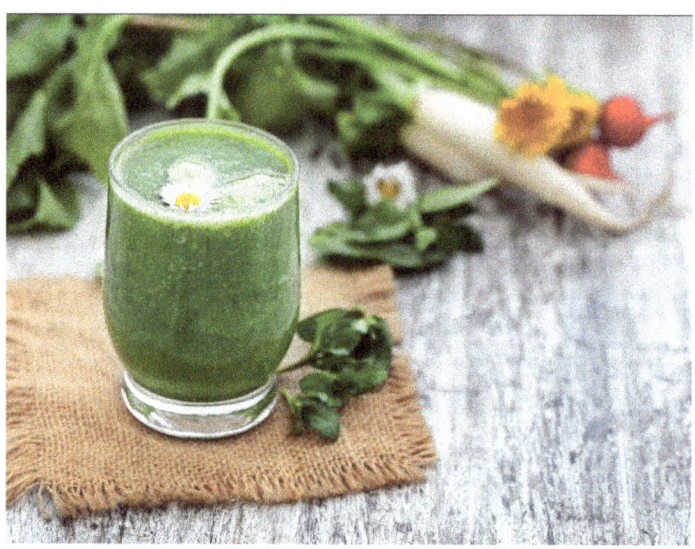

CARROT APHRODISIAC POWER

Not only is this juice a powerful aphrodisiac, but it is also an amazing antioxidant. Drink it on a regular basis to make sure you are always full of energy. Maca powder is optional.

Serves-2

Ingredients:

- 4 carrots
- 2 celery sticks
- 4 big apples
- 1 cucumber
- 2 kiwis
- 1 lime
- Maca powder to spice up
- 1 small piece of ginger

Instructions:

1. Blend all the ingredients

2. Add maca powder and stir well.

3. Serve immediately.

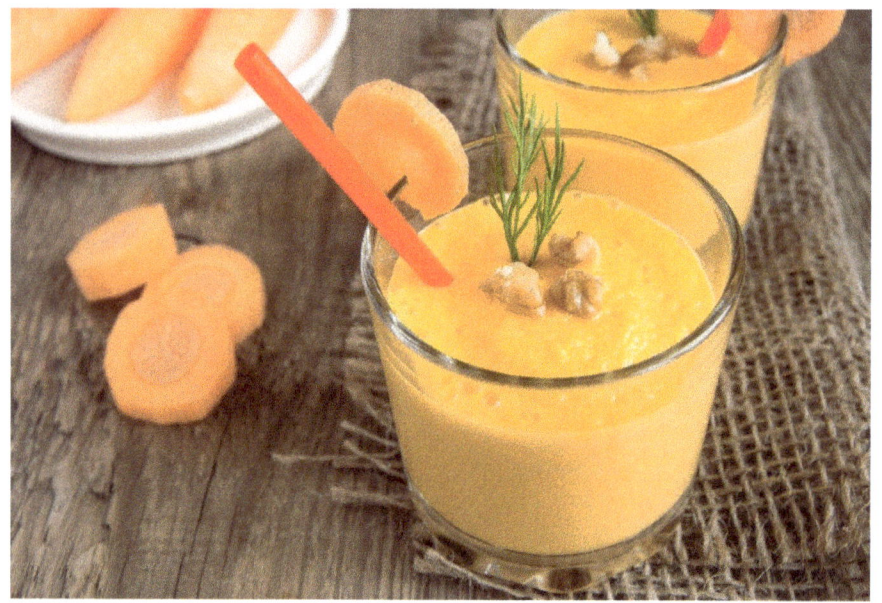

Chapter 4 Aphrodisiac Herbs

Some of nature's herbs can get you in the mood for love. Herbal aphrodisiacs have been used by both men and women for centuries with the belief that it can stimulate and strengthen their sex lives. Both the Romans and the Egyptians are known for brewing amorous herbs as love elixirs. They loved creating their own rituals.

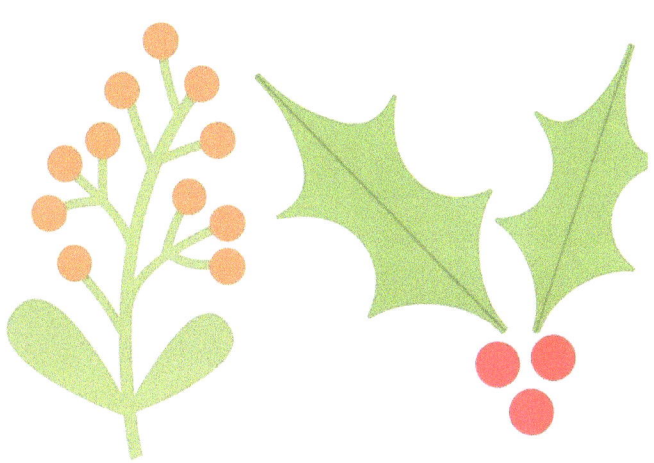

Unfortunately, our times are different and oftentimes too fast-paced. We are stressed out, lack energy and time, and usually indulge in foods that are bad for us. Herbs offer a myriad of natural solutions to get back on a healthy track and discover a new, healthy and more sexually fit version of yourself. Of course, remember that it's not only about using some herbs. Herbs can help you have more energy so that you can make a conscious decision to take better care of your body and mind. Physical fitness means better sex; there is no doubt about it. Rebalance yourself with herbs and get back on a healthy track like you deserve.

The knowledge of traditional herbs is used to stimulate desire and sensitivity in love making. Here are some of the best aphrodisiac herbs for both men and women.

Make sure you consult your physician before you get started on the herbal treatments mentioned in this chapter. This is of paramount importance, especially if you are on medication, have recently undergone surgery or are just about to undergo one. The same applies when you are pregnant/lactating or with any serious health condition.

Many herbs can interact with medical prescriptions. Always consult with your doctor before using. Avoid prolonged intake. Before purchasing herbs, research the brand first. Avoid extremely cheap products that very often don't meet basic safety standards and can be bad for your health. My wife and I usually visit health/organic food stores and herbal stores.

Familiarize yourself with this chapter and choose one remedy at a time to see if it works for you. Avoid mixing too many herbs. It's better to choose one, to see if it works for you and your partner. The herbs can be consumed as herbal infusions as well as capsules and tablets (perfect solution for busy people). You can also use powdered supplements and have them in your smoothies or water (just like I suggested with maca and guarana).

Ashwagandha (also called: Indian, Ayurvedic Genseng). MALE AND FEMALE APHRODISIAC.

- Ashwagandha is also known as the Indian Ginseng and

is used to increase overall physical stamina and health.

- It has an invigorating effect on the nervous system. It works as a mild antidepressant and is also used to treat anxiety and insomnia.

- It increases concentration.

- It reduces inflammation.

- It acts as a tonic and stimulates the immune system.

- It is a natural stress fighter and mood enhancer.

- Females can use it to alleviate menstrual problems.

- Finally, and most importantly for us, it is a natural aphrodisiac and it is even used to treat male and female fertility problems. Pretty multifunctional herb, right? Well, there is more...

- It can be also applied topically to help treat wounds and skin problems.

- Overall a really amazing, anti-age, holistic, natural herb.

Predications (important)

- Avoid prolonged treatments with Ashwagandha, unless under guidance of your health professional.

- Avoid if you suffer from low or high blood pressure, stomach ulcers, diabetes and thyroid disorders.

- Not recommended for pregnant/lactating women.

- It may interact with medical drugs such as sedative medications as well as medications that increase the immune system (since Ashwagandha has the same effect, when combined with another drug, even natural, it can actually cause the opposite effect and decrease the immune system).

Ginko biloba (MALE APHRODISIAC)

- Ginko has originated in Asia and is a popular herb used in different products.

- It is traditionally used to improve memory and concentration.

- It is also used in ophthalmology as it can help treat various eye conditions such as glaucoma and diabetic eye disease (avoid self-medication though, especially if you suffer from any serious eye condition like the above-mentioned)

- It can help alleviate headaches and vertigo.

- As an aphrodisiac, the consumption of Ginko increases blood circulation which can help men with erectile dysfunction.

IMPORTANT PREUCATIONS:

- Never use it if you are on any medication that slows blood clotting (ibuprofen is one of them).

- Avoid if you suffer from diabetes.

- If you are a female trying to get pregnant, this herb may slow down and even inhibit the process.

- It can seriously interfere with liver medications. Avoid.

- It may cause allergic reactions in some people.

- Do not use before, during and after recovering from surgery (consult your physician)

Horny Goat Weed (also called *yin yang huo* in TCM)

- As the name implies, this herb is known to stimulate

sexual desire and improve male fertility. Horny goat weed is a very powerful aphrodisiac and should be used with caution.

- It is also used to improve memory, reduce stress and help recover after disease.

- It strengthens the bones and is used in natural osteoporosis treatments. It is also used for joint pain and physical fatigue.

- It is recommended as a male aphrodisiac. Not only does it enhance sexual desire, but it also helps you last longer in bed and is used to treat erectile problems.

- Recommended for women going through menopause (as well as after) as it helps strengthen the bones.

PREUCATIONS:

- Avoid if on any standard or natural liver medications. Since this herb is also used on liver treatments, your body may rebel and the opposite reaction may occur.

- Avoid if you suffer from low blood pressure.

- Stay on the safe side, and avoid using when pregnant/lactating.

Muira Puama (male and female aphrodisiac)

- Muira Puama is known as a potency wood that increases psychological and physical aspects of sexual function.

- It is also helpful in relieving stress and for toning the nervous system which makes it a perfect aphrodisiac for a busy, stressed out MODERN person.

- Females can use it to alleviate menstrual cramps and irregular periods.

- It also increases elasticity of the joints and reduces inflammation.

Precautions:

Little is known whether this herb is safe to use by pregnant and lactating women. No possible side effect information had been found, however if you suffer from any serious medical condition, please suggest your physician before using. Better safe than sorry, right?

Cordyceps (male aphrodisiac)

- Cordyceps is one of the most sought after Chinese herbal, natural, and anti-aging medicines.

- It has a wide range of therapeutic benefits which include longevity and sexual enhancement.

- It is used for respiratory tract problems and immune system disorders.

- Some researchers say that this natural remedy is so powerful that it can even cure cancer.

- Used in all kinds of recoveries to strengthen the body and mind.

PREUCATIONS:

- Not recommended for pregnant or lactating women

- If you suffer from any serious auto immune system condition consult with your physician before using, especially if you are already on medication. Even though this natural remedy is a natural immune system booster, too much of it (especially when combined with other treatments) can have an opposite effect and decrease the immune system which can be detrimental to your health.

Rhodiola Rosea (male and female aphrodisiac)

- Rhodiola Rosea improves the level of serotonin and dopamine in the body which reduces the stress levels as well as increases physical and sexual performance.

- It acts as a natural mental and physical stimulant strengthening the immune system.

- It is used to lower cholesterol levels and to detoxify the body.

- Commonly used by athletes to improve their performance (and improve your performance - in the bedroom!)

PREUCATIONS:

It is generally considered safe, especially when used for no longer than 6 weeks (The treatment can be repeated only after you take a break).

Again, if you suffer from any serious health condition, seek professional medical advice to stay on the safe side.

Certain aphrodisiac herbs can stimulate sexual desire in females and help them embrace their sensuality. These are especially useful for women!

Brazilian Catuba (male and female)

- Catuba is used in tonics to strengthen the nervous system. This herb is said to produce erotic dreams and increase the libido.

- As an additional benefit, catuba is also effective against viruses.

- Tonic and immune system stimulator

PREUCATIONS:

- It may interact with certain medications for low blood pressure and immune systems. Consult your physician before use.

- Avoid if pregnant or lactating.

Clavo huasca (male and female aphrodisiac)

- Clavo huasca stimulates libido and improves the sexual function for women.

- It is an extremely strong sexual stimulant that is said to be the remedy for female frigidity caused by past traumas and stress.

- Other uses: tonic, natural pain reliever, muscle relaxant, digestive stimulant, immune system booster

- It also works as male aphrodisiac for erectile dysfunction.

PRECAUTIONS:

This natural remedy is commonly used in South America but very little scientific research has been done so far. It is considered to be generally safe, if a person is not on medication nor suffering from any serious health condition. However, one should abstain from prolonged uses. I suggest you consult your physician first to keep on the safe side.

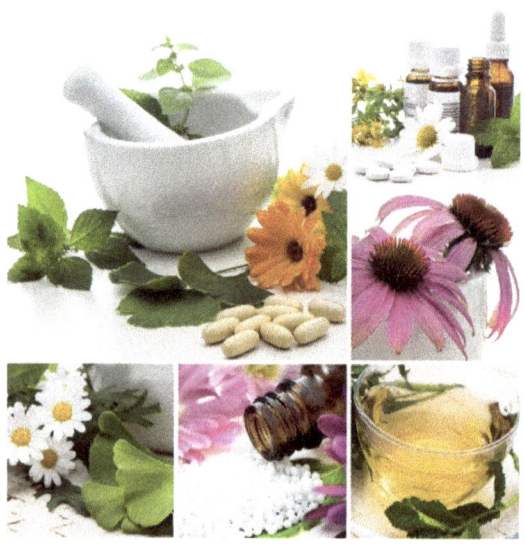

Damiana (male and female aphrodisiac)

- Damiana has a reputation for being an erotic herb and it can help women who find it difficult to achieve orgasm because of anxiety and depression.

- Damiana is known to produce short lived euphoric state.

- It is also used for headaches, nervous stomach, digestive problems caused

   by stress as well as chronic constipation.

PREUCATIONS:

- Use with caution especially if you suffer from high blood pressure.

- Large doses may cause too much euphoria and increased heart beat.

- If you suffer from diabetes, make sure you consult with your physician first (Damiana may affect blood sugar levels and even interact with some medications).

- Avoid in pregnancy

Guarana (male and female aphrodisiac)

- I have already mentioned it with my recipes: guarana stimulates the movement of energy in the body and boosts blood circulation in women.

- It is also used to prolong sexual endurance both for men and women.

- Used by athletes.

- Recommended for weight loss treatments as well as periods of fatigue and exhaustion.

PREUCATIONS:

- Avoid if you are caffeine sensitive, suffer from high blood pressure, or are pregnant and lactating.

- Most resources also recommend avoiding guarana during menstruation (it may increase the blood flow).

- Avoid before, during and after surgery (consult with your doctor)

Maca (male and female, but especially female!)

- This one is an aphrodisiac classic and it is really easy to get in health food stores. You may have noticed that many of my recipes use it!

- Maca can help the body adjust to the stress of modern living acting as a natural energy booster.

- As an aphrodisiac, it helps to balance hormones to increase libido.

- For women, maca can help normalize the menstrual cycle and stimulate fertility. It is also recommended to reduce the symptoms of menopause.

- My wife used to be a big coffee addict. Coffee led her to adrenal exhaustion. Maca helped her switch to juices, smoothies and herbal infusions.

- It is also used in osteoporosis treatments as well as to strengthen the immune system.

PRECAUTIONS:

- Avoid maca if you have any medical condition that might be made worse by exposure to estrogen.

- Not enough medical research has been done to confirm whether maca is safe in pregnancy and breast-feeding. I suggest you consult your physician to stay on the safe side.

Shatavari (female aphrodisiac)

- It is a well-known Ayurvedic remedy that works as an aphrodisiac by bringing sexual balance into a woman's life.

- It can also alleviate menopausal symptoms and regulate sexual hormones.

- Other uses include: relieving digestive problems, headaches, PMS, hormonal imbalances, menopause problems, and uterine bleeding.

- It is used to stimulate milk production in women.

- It is also a great antioxidant, anti-age and immune system booster. Can help prevent female hair loss due to hormonal imbalances or pregnancy/menopause.

PREUCATIONS:

- It is generally considered safe, but I suggest you consult it with a medical practitioner, naturopath or even better - an Ayurvedic doctor specializing in female health.

- Many researchers recommend avoiding it during pregnancy.

Chapter 5 Aromatherapy and Massage for Lovers

My wife and I are absolutely in love with aromatherapy and we use it every day. Our apartment is full of essential oils and we always experiment with them. We are also big fans of massage.

What is so special about aromatherapy? Well, humans have always used odorous concoctions to increase their appeal to the opposite sex. Perfume bottles that are found in the Egyptian ruins testify to the value people place on aromatherapy since ancient times.

Aromatherapy is a great way to add spice into a relationship. Scents have been used for centuries in sexual rituals and are effective in the art of seduction. Like I said in the previous chapter, our modern world is very stressful. Stress is the number one wellness killer. Many friends of mine confide in me telling me how they lost interest in sex. They are anxious, overloaded with work, and simply don't know how to unwind. Sitting on a sofa watching TV does not help at all! They are in a vicious circle that never seems to end. Moreover, it destroys communication in a relationship.

Regular visits to your local spa, especially with your partner, could do wonders, but...

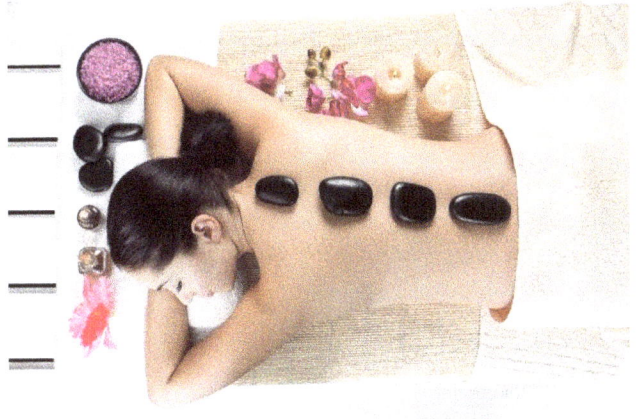

1. Very few people can afford going to spa on a regular basis. Imagine how much money you would spend by using spa services every day or every other day.

2. What's better than your own bedroom? I mean, you can go to spa to relax and even fall asleep when getting a professional massage treatment done. But you can get much more when staying at home. All you need to do is to grasp the basics of aromatherapy. You can treat your partner to massages (at the end of this chapter I will show you how), aromatherapy baths, and you can also use the oils to create an incredibly spicy atmosphere in your apartment. What more do you need?

PREPARATION:

BASE OIL/ VEGETABLE OILS

Since you can't apply essential oils undiluted on your (or your partners) skin (pure essential oils can cause an allergic reaction, rashes and even burn the skin which would spoil the whole fun, right?), you will need to dilute them in a good quality, cold-pressed vegetable oil. These are also called base oils.

Here are some of my suggestions:

- Coconut oil (one of my favorites, it is really amazing and multi functional!)
- Sweet almond oil
- Hazelnut oil
- Argan Oil (great for facials)
- Avocado Oil
- Grape seed oil
- Castor oil (nice but a bit sticky)
- Olive oil (as a last resort you can steal some from your kitchen)

- St John's Wart oil

Here is what you do:

Mix 1 tablespoon of base oil with 4-6 drops of your chosen essential oil to spice things up. You can also mix more than one essential oil, but remember not to overdose the maximum amount of essential oil drops which should be no more than 6 per 1 tablespoon of base oil (there are some exception of course, but for simple massages and home treatments, I suggest you stick to this rule that is recommended for beginners).

IMPORTANT NOTE FOR BEGINNERS:

Oils such as clove, cinnamon, and basil are pretty strong and those who have sensitive skin, may get allergic reactions. I suggest you test your blend on your forearm first. You may want to use weaker blends to start.

The same applies to citrus oils as well as mint.

Better safe than sorry!

Below you will find some of my favorite essential oils that are also known for their aphrodisiac properties. Make sure you get acquainted with possible precautions. Abstain from using them if you are pregnant, lactating, or are on medication (some essential oils are safe in pregnancy; however it is a must to consult your doctor as well as your local aromatherapist. I always say that even with natural stuff, one must learn all possible precautions and stick to the safe side).

After explaining to you all about essential oils that stimulate libido, I will share some of my recipes with you. I hope you will enjoy them!

LIBIDO STIMULATING ESSENTIAL OILS:

Basil Essential Oil

- Basil has an erotic sweet and spicy scent that is associated with love and fertility.

- Basil can awaken the senses and can stimulate lovers' basic sexual instinct.

- It can be used as a massage oil that can help relax and sooth the mind.

- It is helpful for those who suffer from depression. However, it is not recommended for people suffering from clinical depression as it may aggravate their condition.

- Use in small amounts and weaker concentrations, especially if you have sensitive skin that goes red easily.

Bergamot Essential Oil

- Bergamot is an evocative scent that easily improves the mood for lovers.

- It has a lemon and floral aroma that is able to relieve

tension and nervousness.

- Recommended for those who suffer from insomnia and anxiety.

- Avoid direct sun exposure after applying.

Cedarwood Essential Oil

- I recommend cedarwood for lovers who want to deepen their relationship by experiencing a spiritual dimension during love making.

- It is helpful in soothing anxiety and draw lovers into a sensual bliss.

- It helps alleviate tension headaches.

Frankincense Essential Oil

- Frankincense has a memorable aroma that can trigger a deeper awareness in a relationship.

- It is recommended for meditation. It helps connect with the "here and now."

- It can bring more spirituality and mystery to your love

life.

Ginger Essential Oil

- The spicy aroma of ginger is perfect for aromatherapy.
- It effectively increases vitality to ensure a night full of passion.
- It has a nice, warming effect. You can use it to prevent colds and flu.

Jasmine Essential Oil

- Jasmine is best used to rekindle the flame of a former love.
- Its erotic scent promises lasting sexual effect and can bring warmth to a relationship.
- It helps achieve relaxation but is energizing at the same time. It balanced the body and mind connection bringing peace after an argument between lovers.

Juniper Essential Oil

- Juniper can be used to remove negative feelings such as

doubt and insecurity.

- I highly recommend this scent for lovers who are experiencing emotional trouble to help them reestablish their relationship.

- On a physical level, it helps fight water retention and removes the feeling of being tired. It has energizing properties.

- Its smell is herbal and really soft. Great for those who don't like to feel overwhelmed by strong aromatherapy fragrances.

Lavender Essential Oil

- Lavender is an evocative scent that relaxes the body and mind.

- Its soothing aroma is perfect for a sweet and romantic night for lovers.

- Recommended for those who struggle with anxiety, insomnia and high stress levels. Lavender can help unwind.

- Don't use too much of it as you may feel too sleepy!

Lime Essential Oil

- The tangy scent of lime evokes laughter in a romantic union. The scent also increases the desire for passion.

- Use lime to lighten the atmosphere and ease anxiety.

- All citric scents act as anti-depressants and bring more energy, soothing the stressed out minds at the same time. What more can you ask for?

Patchouli Essential Oil

- Patchouli is a sexually provocative scent that removes inhibitions for a sensual romantic experience.

- The deep musky scent of patchouli encourages desire and passion.

- Recommended for women who suffer from frigidity and can't open to sexual relationships due to past traumas or depression.

Rose Absolute Essential Oil

- Rose absolute is an aphrodisiac with healing properties.

- It can uplift emotions and encourages a more open

relationship.

- It is also amazing for the skin. It acts as a natural moisturizer and prevents premature ageing. My wife loves it for facials!

Ylang Ylang Essential Oil

- The scent of ylang ylang is a powerful aphrodisiac that can enhance the attraction between two lovers.

- It can stimulate energy and promote a more sensual experience during sex.

- It is especially recommended as a libido booster for women who lost interest in sex.

- Its smell is really strong and some people may find it too overwhelming. Make sure it works well for you and your partner before you begin to use it for massages.

Essential oils and other natural aromatherapy products offer a myriad of scents to enhance your sexual experience. Make sure you purchase good quality, organic essential oils.

Aromatherapy General Precautions

Aromatherapy is a very safe and easy therapy to use, but keep in mind that there are certain precautions:

- Remember to wash your hands after applying aromatherapy massage

- Do not apply the essential oils in their pure form as they may cause an allergic reaction. Instead, use blends that contain 2-5% essential oils diluted in good-quality cold-pressed oil

-After using citrus oils, like for example lemon, verbena, bergamot, orange etc. avoid direct sun exposure, even up to 8 hours after the treatment

- Do not apply oils after surgery (unless you have consulted with a doctor) or on open wounds or rashes of unknown origin

- Do not use the oils after chemotherapy (unless suggested by a doctor)

- Keep the oils away from the eyes and mucus membranes

- Use the oils only topically (unless you have consulted with an aromatherapist who specializes in phytoaromatherapy)

- Avoid rosemary, thyme, Spanish and common sage, fennel and hyssop if you suffer from high blood pressure

- Do not apply the treatments described in this book on babies or infants. It doesn't mean that aromatherapy can never be used on babies and infants, but extremely low concentrations should be used. Always consult with a medical or naturopathy doctor first

- Make sure that you research the brand, read safety instructions for each individual oil you buy/use and check the expiration date

- Store your blends in dark glass bottles, preferably in a cool, dry and dark place and remember to use within a maximum of one month after mixing.

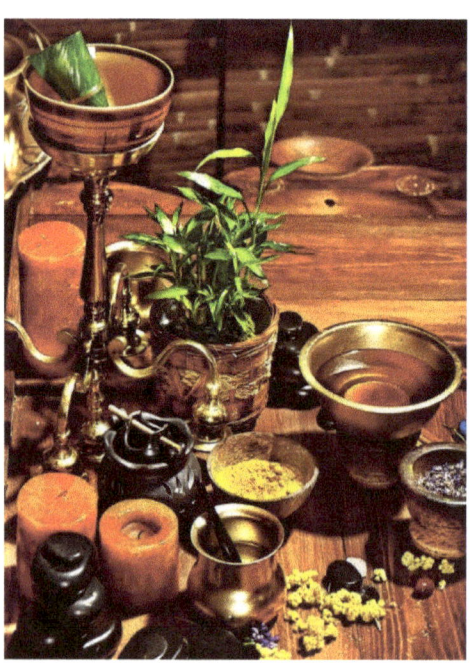

RECIPES

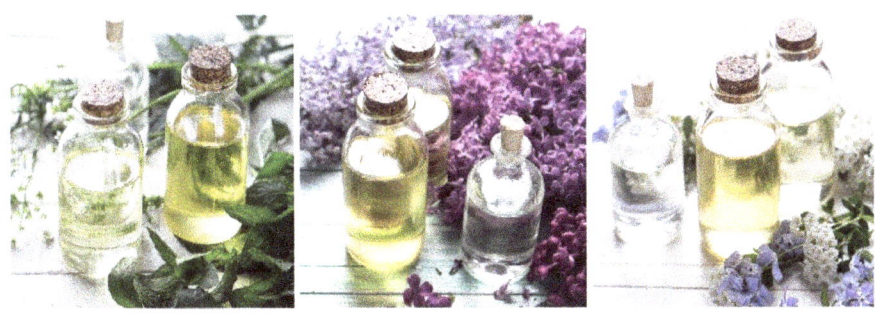

SEXY CLEOPATRA BATH

- 1 cup of warm almond milk
- 2 drops of ylang ylang EO
- 2 drops of lemon EO
- 2 drops of cinamon EO

Stir well before pouring into your bath (make sure that the water is not running and that the temperature is nicely warm). Stir the bath water with your hands before jumping into it.

Super Sensual Mix for HER

- 2 drops of ylang ylang
- 2 drops of bergamot
- 1 tablespoon of coconut oil

Blend and use for sensual all body massage. Focus on the lower back and stomach.

SUPER HOT BLEND FOR HIM

- 3 drops of cinnamon EO
- 3 drops of lavender EO
- 1 tablespoon of coconut oil (or any other base oil that you have at home)

Blend in a mini bowl or a glass and use for an all sensual massage.

SEXY BLEND FOR AMAZINGLY RELAXING FACIAL MASSAGE

Some people find it difficult to relax and unwind. They never stop thinking about their problems and, of course, this can reverberate on their sex life. If your partner is one of those people. Prepare this blend and use it for facial and head massage. It usually does the trick for my nervous wife.

- 1 drop of lavender or lavandin EO
- 1 drop of rose EO
- 1 tablespoon of argan oil

This blend is also great for the skin.

You can use it for head massage, it will soothe the nerves and improve hair condition of your partner, or yours). Head massage is extremely sensual and relaxing!

SUPER WARMING MIX FOR THOSE WHO ARE SHY

- 2 drops of ginger EO
- 2 drops of clove EO
- 2 drops of cinnamon EO
- 2 tablespoons of coconut oil

Mix all the ingredients and use for sensual massage. The reason I suggest you use more base oil in this recipe is that the essential oils mentioned here can be really strong.

Massage Techniques For Lovers

Massage is a great way to improve blood circulation and relieve tension. Romantic massages are also effective in arousing your lover. It is a satisfying way to express intimacy to a partner. Tantric massage is a ritual that helps revitalize sexual energy and is used to awaken the senses. Lovers don't have to be certified massage therapist to be able to provide a great Tantric massage.

- Start of by setting an appropriate mood for love. Dim the lights and use your favorite scents. I also encourage people to warm the room by lighting some candles to make the environment more comfortable.

Begin with the backside

- Add two tablespoon of oil into your hands then rub to warm up the oil. Place your hand on your lovers' lower back and begin gliding your hand up to the neck and around the shoulders. Bring the hand to the lower back and gently kneed the buttocks.

The hand slide

Place the hand parallel to each other and move the hands along the length of the body. Massage all the way down to the buttocks before moving the hands to the neck and shoulders. Ask your lover for feedback on which part of their body feels more sensitive.

Pull-ups

Alternate hand strokes at the side of your lover's body. Place your hands on your partner's hips and gently pull up towards the spine. Remember to do both sides.

Kneading

Stimulate your lover by squeezing their back and buttocks between your thumb and fingers. Alternate squeezing with one hand followed by the other. The fleshy parts of the body can withstand more pressure so you can squeeze these areas a little harder.

Feather stroke

Caress your lover's neck, shoulder, arms and back by lightly brushing your fingertips in feather strokes for at least five minutes. Gently scratch the skin using your fingernails.

Foot caress

Add more oil when necessary in any parts of the process. Repeat the hand slide technique to your lover's thighs and calf. Follow with kneading motions then do the feathery stroke. Concentrate on one leg at a time. Take one foot and cover it generously with oil. Spread it around the ankles and heels. Use the palm of your hands to slide over the foot. Gently rotate each toe and slither the forefinger between them.

Turn over

Continue the massage by turning your lover over and focusing on the chest and stomach. Tease their nipples by gently tracing circles around it. Squeeze a lot of oil on top of the belly button then spread the oil by sliding the hand all over the stomach. Be very gentle around the female breast. Male chest can withstand greater pressure.

Men and women who are receiving tantric massages can experience rise and fall in their sexual energy. These peaks are very sensual and erotic. The main essence of massage for lovers is to heighten their senses and increase sexual attraction for each other.

Did you remember to get your free gift?

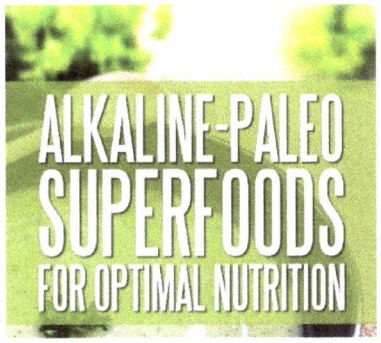

It's waiting for you at:

www.holisticwellnessbooks.com/bonus

Problems with your download?

Contact us: elenajamesbooks@gmail.com

We're here to help.

Conclusion

Do not look at your partner as merely an object of desire. You need to make use of your touch and smell to get intimate with your partner, both physically and emotionally. Doing this will bring you an immense level of satisfaction, while prolonging the sexual performance of you and your partner.

Sex should never be performed just to satisfy your partner's sexual desire. In a situation, where you feel unsatisfied by your partner, you need to communicate this effectively with him or her. Discuss arousal techniques or try different sex positions as per Kamasutra to make the intercourse more enjoyable.

Finally, if you enjoyed this short read, I would love to hear from you in the review section. It's you I am writing for and your feedback would be greatly appreciated.

Thank you and the best of luck,

James Adler

RESOURCES

You will find more books to help you live a healthier lifestyle at:

www.YourWellnessBooks.com

www.ingramcontent.com/pod-product-compliance
Lightning Source LLC
Chambersburg PA
CBHW040947110526
R18273800001B/R182738PG44587CBX00001B/1